52 Headache and Migraine Solutions:

52 Meal Recipes That Will Stop the Pain and Suffering Fast and Effectively

By

Joe Correa CSN

COPYRIGHT

ACKNOWLEDGEMENTS

This book is dedicated to my friends and family that have had mild or serious illnesses so that you may find a solution and make the necessary changes in your life.

52 Headache and Migraine Solutions:

52 Meal Recipes That Will Stop the Pain and Suffering Fast and Effectively

By

Joe Correa CSN

CONTENTS

ABOUT THE AUTHOR

After years of Research, I honestly believe in the positive effects that proper nutrition can have over the body and mind. My knowledge and experience has helped me live healthier throughout the years and which I have shared with family and friends. The more you know about eating and drinking healthier, the sooner you will want to change your life and eating habits.

Nutrition is a key part in the process of being healthy and living longer so get started today. The first step is the most important and the most significant.

INTRODUCTION

52 Headache and Migraine Solutions: 52 Meal Recipes That Will Stop the Pain and Suffering Fast and Effectively

By Joe Correa CSN

Migraines and headaches are common issues that you must have experienced at least once in your life. There are so many different factors that cause and contribute towards migraines. But before I get to that, let's make one thing clear – there is a big difference between migraines and headaches.

A typical migraine feeling makes you think your head is about to explode out of a throbbing pain. Symptoms like neck pain, lack of stamina, bad coordination, and loosing concentration are usual migraine side effects. However, if these symptoms are getting stronger every day, you should visit your physician for examination and consultation.

Headaches are not constant like migraines, but they are also painful and can be caused by lack of proper nutrition. Insufficient amounts of magnesium, fiber, calcium, or carbs is one of the main causes for headaches.

Changing some of your eating habits can prevent and even treat these conditions. There are many studies and research that show the connection between headaches and food. Some foods like rice, greens, and fruits have the amazing ability to prevent migraines and headaches.

Besides being amazing for headaches and migraines, these recipes are based on raw and healthy ingredients that will improve your overall health.

I have learned that every individual has his or her own triggers that cause headaches. Some people have bad reactions to certain dairy products, eggs, meat, chocolate, etc., without them being aware that these foods can increase the amount of headaches they will have. However, salmon is known as an omega 3 fatty acid booster, and it's proven to help with inflammation which leads to migraines and headaches.

You should experiment with the food you eat and learn to listen to what your body has to tell you. For example, if you eat large amounts of a certain food and your headache appears, then you should remove it from your diet.

This book offers a collection of general, pain-reducing foods, that will help you deal with this problem. Meat is minimized in the recipes provided because it contributes to a hormonal imbalance which is one of the most significant triggers for headaches and migraines. Whole grains, vegetables, beans, and fruits, on the other hand, are a perfect choice for your daily diet. You will find all the necessary vitamins, minerals, and other nutrients in every one of these recipes which are a perfect start for a well-balanced diet and a new life without headaches and migraines.

52 HEADACHE AND MIGRAINE SOLUTIONS: 52 MEAL RECIPES THAT WILL STOP THE PAIN AND SUFFERING FAST AND EFFECTIVELY

1. Polenta with Baked Veggies

Ingredients:

1 medium-sized cauliflower head, cut into bite-sized pieces

1 small onion, chopped

1 small butternut squash, peeled and chopped

1 cup of cornmeal

1 garlic clove, minced

2 tbsp of coconut oil, melted

½ tsp of vegetable seasoning mix

¼ tsp of salt

¼ tsp of black pepper, ground

1 tbsp of butter

4 cups of water

Preparation:

Preheat the oven to 475°F.

Combine garlic, onion, cauliflower, and butternut squash in a large bowl. Melt the coconut oil and stir into this mixture. Sprinkle with vegetable seasoning mix, salt, and pepper to taste. Give it a good stir.

Transfer the mixture to a large baking dish. Spread evenly and put it in the oven. Bake for 40 minutes or until vegetables are fork-tender. Stir few times during baking process.

Meanwhile, pour the water into a large non-stick skillet over a medium-high temperature. Bring it to a boil and add cornmeal. Stir in the butter and sprinkle with a pinch of salt to taste. Stir constantly for 1 minute. Reduce the heat to low and cook for 40 minutes, or until nicely creamy polenta.

Transfer polenta to a serving plate and top with baked vegetables.

Serve warm.

Nutrition information per serving: Kcal: 329, Protein: 4.2g, Carbs: 43.6g, Fats: 14.5g

2. Grapefruit Broccoli Smoothie

Ingredients:

1 cup of broccoli, halved

1 medium-sized banana, sliced

½ grapefruit, peeled and chopped

1 tbsp of sesame seeds

1 cup of water

Preparation:

Combine all ingredients in a food processor. Blend until smooth mixture and transfer to a serving glasses. Refrigerate 30 minutes before serving.

Nutrition information per serving: Kcal: 265, Protein: 7.4g, Carbs: 55.3g, Fats: 6.7g

3. Potato Casserole

Ingredients:

6 large potatoes, peeled and halved

2 cups of broccoli, halved

1 cup of cheddar cheese, shredded

1 cup of green onions, chopped

1 tbsp of olive oil

¼ tsp of salt

¼ tsp of black pepper, ground

Preparation:

Preheat the oven to a 350°F.

Place the potatoes in a large pot of boiling water. Cook until fork-tender and remove from the heat. Remove from the heat and drain. Leave it to cool for 10 minutes. in a separate pot, place the broccoli into a boiling process and cook until soften. Remove from the heat and drain. Set aside.

Halve the potatoes and place them into a greased baking dish. Now, make another layer with halved broccoli. Top with shredded cheese and put it in the oven. Bake for 25 minutes. remove from the oven and sprinkle with chopped spring onions. Leave it to cool for few minutes and cut into desired portions.

Nutrition information per serving: Kcal: 351, Protein: 13.2g, Carbs: 60.7g, Fats: 6.4g

4. Garbanzo Salad

Ingredients:

2 cups of garbanzo beans, pre-cooked

2 cups of kidney beans, pre-cooked

3 cups of Iceberg lettuce, shredded

1 large tomato, chopped

1 medium-sized cucumber, sliced

1 small avocado, peeled, pitted and chopped

1 cup of yogurt, fat free

1 garlic clove, crushed

¼ tsp of cumin, ground

Preparation:

Place garbanzo and kidney beans in a pot of boiling water. Cook until soften. Remove from the heat and let it cool for a while.

Now, combine beans, tomato, and cucumber in a large salad bowl. Set aside.

Meanwhile, combine avocado, yogurt, cumin, and garlic in a food processor. Blend until smooth and drizzle over the salad.

Place a handfull of shredded lettuce on a serving plate and top with 2-3 tablespoons of previously made salad.

Serve immedieately.

Nutrition information per serving: Kcal: 171, Protein: 8.6g, Carbs: 28.8g, Fats: 3.7g

5. Oven Baked Rice with Spring Onions

Ingredients:

2 cups of long grain rice

4 tbsp of extra virgin olive oil

1 tsp of salt

3 whole eggs

5 spring onions, finely chopped

½ tsp of black pepper, freshly ground

Preparation:

Preheat the oven to 350°F.

Use a package instructions to prepare the rice. Set aside.

In a medium-sized skillet heat up two tablespoons of olive oil and add onions. Stir fry for 3-4 minutes. Meanwhile, beat the eggs and pour into skillet. Cook for two minutes, remove from the heat and combine with rice.

Spread the remaining oil in a small casserole dish. Add rice mixture, sald, and pepper. Bake for 20 minutes.

Serve warm.

Instead of oven, you can prepare this dish in a large wok pan. Simply stir-fry the cooked rice until lightly crispy. Serve.

Nutrition information per serving: Kcal: 409, Protein: 8.9g, Carbs: 60g, Fats: 14.3g

6. Watermelon Salad

Ingredients:

6 cups of watermelon, cut into bite-sized pieces

2 tbsp of balsamic vinegar

½ small red onion, sliced

1 tbsp of fresh mint, roughly chopped

½ tsp of salt

Preparation:

Place the onion into a medium pot. Pour water enough to cover it and add a pinch of salt. Set aside for 15 minutes. Drain well and transfer to a large salad bowl.

Add watermelon chops and drizzle with vinegar. Give it a good stir and top with fresh mint leaves.

Nutrition information per serving: Kcal: 53, Protein: 0.9g, Carbs: 12.5g, Fats: 0.3g

7. Poached Salmon

Ingredients:

1 lb of wild salmon fillets, skinless and boneless

1 tbsp of fresh dill, finely chopped

1 large onion, sliced

2 small carrots, sliced

2 tbsp of lemon juice

2 bay leaves

4 cups of water

Preparation:

Preheat the oven to 350°F.

Pour water in a large skillet. Bring it to a boil and add dill, carrots, onion, lemon juice, and bay leaves. Cook for about 2-3 minutes and remove from the heat. Set aside.

Meanwhile, place the salmon fillets into a large baking sheet. Pour the previosly prepared liquid. Cover with a lid and place it in the oven. Bake for 20 minutes, or until set. Remove from the heat and leave it to cool for a while.

Serve.

Nutrition information per serving: Kcal: 239, Protein: 24.5g, Carbs: 6.3g, Fats: 5.2g

8. Ginger Dates Smoothie

Ingredients:

1 cup of spinach, chopped

½ medium-sized avocado, pitted, peeled, and cubed

3 dates, pitted and chopped

1 tbsp of lemon juice

1 tbsp of fresh ginger, grated

Preparation:

Combine all ingredients in a food processor. Blend until nicely smooth. Transfer to a serving glasses and refrigerate for 15 minutes. For extra thickness, refrigerate more.

Nutrition information per serving: Kcal: 389, Protein: 5.2g, Carbs: 48.8g, Fats: 21.2g

9. Warm Broccoli Soup

Ingredients:

2oz fresh broccoli

2oz Brussel sprouts

A handful of fresh parsley, finely chopped

1 tsp of dry thyme

1 tbsp of fresh lemon juice

¼ tsp of sea salt

Preparation:

Place the broccoli in a deep pot and pour enough water to cover. Bring it to a boil and cook until tender. Remove from the heat and drain.

Transfer to a food processor. Add fresh parsley, thyme, and about 1 cup of water. Pulse until smooth mixture. Return to a pot and add some more water. Bring it to a boil and cook for several minutes, over a minimum temperature. Season with salt and add fresh lemon juice. Serve warm.

Nutrition information per serving: Kcal: 50, Protein: 3.7g, Carbs: 9.9g, Fats: 0.6g

10. Stuffed Tomatoes

Ingredients:

10 oz of spinach, chopped

4 medium-sized tomatoes

½ cup of Mozzarella cheese, crumbled

½ cup of Parmesan cheese, grated

1 small onion, finely chopped

2 tbsp of fresh parsley, finely chopped

¼ tsp of salt

¼ tsp of black pepper, ground

Preparation:

Preheat the oven to 350°F.

Place spinach in a pot of boiling water. Cook for 2 minutes, or until soften. Remove from the heat and drain well. Set aside.

Hollow the tomatoes and reserve the pulp. Chop it into a small pieces and add it to spinach. Stir in the cheeses and toss well to combine. Spoon in the mixture into tomatoes.

Place stuffed tomatoes in a large baking sheet. Place it in the oven and bake for about 6-7 minutes. remove from the heat and leave it to cool for a while.

Nutrition information per serving: Kcal: 159, Protein: 13.2g, Carbs: 15.6g, Fats: 7.3g

11. Brown Rice Mushroom Risotto

Ingredients:

1 cup of brown rice

1 cup of button mushrooms, sliced

½ medium-sized onion, finely chopped

3 spring onions, sliced

3 tbsp of extra virgin olive oil

½ tsp of salt

1 tsp of dry marjoram

Preparation:

Place the rice in a deep pot. Add 2 cups of water and bring it to a boil. Reduce the heat and cook until the water evaporates. Stir occasionally. Set aside.

Heat up one tablespoon of olive oil over a medium-high heat. Add chopped onion and stir-fry for 3-4 minutes, stirring constantly. Now add the mushrooms and continue to cook until the water evaporates.

Stir in the remaining olive oil, rice, spring onions, salt, and marjoram. Add one cup of water and continue to cook for another 10 minutes.

Serve warm.

Nutrition information per serving: Kcal: 243, Protein: 16.4g, Carbs: 24.5g, Fats: 11.3g

12. Peanut Butter Smoothie

Ingredients:

1 medium-sized banana, sliced

½ cup of Greek yogurt

1 tbsp of cinnamon, ground

1 tbsp of peanut butter

1 tbsp of coconut flour

Preparation:

Combine all ingredients in a food processor. Blend all until smooth mixture. Transfer to a serving glass and refrigrate for 1 hour before serving.

Nutrition information per serving: Kcal: 216, Protein: 5.6g, Carbs: 35.6g, Fats: 8.5g

13. Black Beans & Squash Stew

Ingredients:

1 medium-sized buternut squash, peeled and chopped

4 cups of black beans, canned

4 large tomatoes, blended

1 small onion, sliced

1 garlic clove, minced

4 medium-sized bell peppers, chopped

1 tsp of cumin, ground

1 tsp of dried oregano, minced

1 tbsp of olive oil

¼ tsp of black pepper, ground

¼ tsp of salt

Preparation:

Place squash in a pot of boiling water and cook for 10 minutes, or until fork-tender. Drain well and set aside.

Preheat the oil in a large pot over a medium-high temperature. Add onions and stir-fry for 5 minutes, or until translucent. Add beans, garlic, peppers, cumin, and oregano and stir.

Meanwhile, place tomatoes in a food processor and blend until smooth mixture. Transfer to a pot and give it a good stir. Bring to a boil and reduce the heat to low. Add squash, stir once, and cover with a lid. Cook for about 20-25 minutes and remove from the heat. Sprinkle with some salt and pepper to taste.

Serve warm.

Nutrition information per serving: Kcal: 201, Protein: 8.2g, Carbs: 40.3g, Fats: 3.7g

14. Curry Veggies Salad

Ingredients:

1 lb of broccoli, halved

1 cup of sour cream, fat-free

2 large tomatoes, wedged

1 tsp of curry powder

¼ tsp of dry mustard

½ cup of skim milk

5 Romaine lettuce leaves

Preparation:

Place broccoli in a pot of boiling water and cook until soften. Remove from the heat and drain well. Transfer to a serving bowl and set aside to cool for 5 minutes.

Meanwhile, combine, milk, sour cream, curry, and mustard in a mixing bowl. Toss well to combine and pour over the broccoli. Add tomato wedges and stir well.

Place lettuce leaves on a serving plate and spoon the salad onto it. Refrigerate for 2 hours to allow flavors to mingle.

Nutrition information per serving: Kcal: 109, Protein: 3.8g, Carbs: 11.4g, Fats: 2.2g

15. Brown Rice Pudding with Raspberries and Chia Seeds

Ingredients:

¾ cup of brown rice

1 cup of rice milk

¼ cup of honey

1 tbsp of almond butter

¼ tsp of salt

½ cup of raspberries

¼ cup of walnuts

2 tbsp of chia seeds

Preparation:

Bring 2 cups of water to a boil. Add rice and reduce the heat. Cover and cook for about 15 minutes.

Now add one cup of rice milk, honey, almond butter, and salt. Continue to cook for five more minutes. Remove from the heat and cool for a while.

Top with fresh raspberries, walnuts, and chia seeds. Serve.

Nutrition information per serving: Kcal: 240, Protein: 5.7g, Carbs: 36.7g, Fats: 8.4g

16. Crispy Cauliflower Sliders

Ingredients:

1 cup of fresh button mushrooms

3 tbsp of flax seeds plus 9 tbsp of water

¾ cup of chia seeds

¾ cup of brown rice

¾ cup of buckwheat bread crumbs

1 tsp of tarragon

1 tsp of parsley

1 tsp of garlic powder

1 cup of chopped spinach

Preparation:

Pour 1 cup of water in a small saucepan. Bring it to boil and cook rice until it's slightly sticky. This should take about 10 minutes.

At the same time, cook chia seeds until soft in a separate pot. Finely chop mushrooms. Thoroughly rinse spinach.

Mix all the ingredients together in a large bowl. Put the bowl into the fridge to chill for 15 to 30 minutes.

Take mixture out of the fridge and form into patties. Make sure cooking surfaces are cleaned and greased before adding patties to prevent them from sticking. Fry each piece on a medium temperature for about 5 minutes on both side.

Nutrition information per serving: Kcal: 220, Protein: 6.1g, Carbs: 40.1g, Fats: 3.6g

17. Tomato Strawberry Smoothie

Ingredients:

½ cantaloupe, peeled and chopped

1 cup of orange juice

1 cup of strawberries, halved

1 medium-sized tomato, chopped

Preparation:

Combine all ingredients in a blender. Add few ice cubes and blend until nicely smooth. Transfer to a serving glass and serve immediately!

Nutrition information per serving: Kcal: 253, Protein: 5.3g, Carbs: 62.4g, Fats: 1.2g

18. Ginger Quinoa Porridge

Ingredients:

1/2 cup of orange juice

1 tsp of fresh ginger, grated

½ cup of dates, pitted and chopped

1 cup of white quinoa, pre-cooked

½ cup of dried apricots, chopped

1 tsp of fresh orange zest, grated

1 tsbp of toasted almonds, chopped

¼ tsp of cinnamon, ground

Preparation:

Place quinoa in a pot of boiling water. Cook for 3 minutes and reduce the heat to low. Cook for another 10 minutes or until soften and fluffy. Add all other ingredients except almonds and give it a good stir. Remove from the heat and set aside for 10 minutes to cool. Top with chopped almonds and serve.

Nutrition information per serving: Kcal: 171, Protein: 5.2g, Carbs: 32.5g, Fats: 4.7g

19. Creamy Pumpkin Soup

Ingredients:

3 lbs of pumpkin, peeled and cubed

2 small onions, sliced

5 cups of chicken broth

2 cups of skim milk

3 tbsp of Greek yogurt

2 tbsp of pumpkin seeds

1 garlic clove, minced

1 tsp of vegetable oil

¼ tsp of salt

¼ tsp of black pepper, ground

Preparation:

Preheat the oil in a large nonstick saucepan over a medium-high temperature. Add onions and stir-fry until soften. Add vegetable broth, pumpkin cubes, milk, sage, and garlic. Bring it to a boil and reduce the heat to low. Cover with a lid and cook for 35 minutes. Remove from the heat and set aside to cool for 10 minutes.

Transfer the mixture into a food processor. Blend until nicely creamy mixture. Transfer to a serving bowl or previously used saucepan. Add a pinch of salt and pepper to taste and stir well.

Serve warm.

Nutrition information per serving: Kcal: 191, Protein: 4.3g, Carbs: 27.7g, Fats: 4.1g

20. Nutmeg Fruit Smoothie

Ingredients:

2 large oranges, peeled and wedged

2 medium-sized apples, wedged

1 small mango, peeled, pitted and chopped

1 small carrot, sliced

½ tsp of nutmeg

1 tsp of cinnamon, ground

1 tbsp of honey

½ cup of water

Preparation:

Combine all ingredients in a food processor. Blend until smooth and transfer to a serving glasses. Refrigerate 30 minutes before serving.

Nutrition information per serving: Kcal: 316, Protein: 3.6g, Carbs: 79.5g, Fats: 1.8g

21. Zuchini Lasagna

Ingredients:

1 medium-sized zuchinni, peeled and chopped

2 oz of Parmesan cheese, grated

2 oz of cottage cheese, crumbled

2 oz of Mozarella cheese, grated

8 oz of lasagna noodles, pre-cooked

2 cups of tomato sauce

1 small onion, sliced

1 garlic clove, minced

¼ tsp of oregano, ground

2 tsp of dried basil, ground

½ tsp of Cayenne pepper, ground

¼ tsp of salt

Preparation:

Preheat the oven to 370 °F.

Place zucchini in a pot of boiling water. Cook until fork-tender and remove from the heat to cool for 5 minutes. Drain well and slice into small bite-sized pieces. Set aside.

Combine all cheeses in a mixing bowl. Pour in the tomato sauce and stir well.

Grease a large baking dish with some oil. Spread the cheese and tomato mixture and make a first layer. Now, add one layer of noodles, then one layer of zucchini slices.Repeat layering process until left out of ingredients. Add some extra cheese and 1 tablespoon of tomato sauce on top. Sprinkle with Cayenne pepper for extra flavor.

Cover with foil and put it in the oven. Bake for 30 minutes and remove from the oven to cool.

Cut into portions and serve warm.

Nutrition information per serving: Kcal: 275, Protein: 18.3g, Carbs: 41.3g, Fats: 5.4g

22. Leafy Detox Smoothie

Ingredients:

¼ cup of roasted almonds, finely chopped

¼ cup of baby spinach, finely chopped

¼ cup of arugula

1 tbsp of almond butter

½ tsp of ground turmeric

1 cup of rice milk

A handful of ice cubes

Preparation:

Toss all the ingredients in a blender. Pulse to combine.

Nutrition information per serving: Kcal: 181, Protein: 4.6g, Carbs: 17.1g, Fats: 11.5g

23. Turkey & Mushrooms Stew

Ingredients:

1 lb of turkey breasts, skinless and boneless

5 oz of button mushrooms, chopped

2 garlic cloves, minced

1 tbsp of fresh parsley, finely chopped

1 tbsp of honey, raw

½ tsp of salt

¼ tsp of black pepper, ground

Preparation:

Combine all ingredients except honey in a slow cooker. Pour water enough to cover all ingredients. Cover with a lid and cook for 7 hours. Remove from the heat and let it stand for 20 minutes. Open the lid and let it cool for 10 minutes and then stir in honey.

Nutrition information per serving: Kcal: 116, Protein: 16.5g, Carbs: 8.8g, Fats: 1.7g

24. Quinoa Muffins

Ingredients:

1.5 cups of quinoa flour

0.5 cup of buckwheat flour

3 tbsp of almond butter

1 cup of almond milk

½ cup of honey

1 tsp of baking powder

½ tsp of salt

2 tbsp of raw cocoa

2 tbsp of flax seed plus 6 tbsp of water

1 tsp organic vanilla extract

1 tsp lemon zest

Preparation:

Preheat oven to 325 degrees. Line one 6-cup muffin tins with paper liners.

Combine all dry ingredients in a large bowl. Gently whisk in almond milk, almond butter, and beat well on high. Add flax seed, water, lemon zest, and reduce the speed to low. Continue beating until well incorporated.

Using a spoon or ice cream scoop, divide the mixture evenly among the tins. Bake for 20-30 or until the toothpick inserted into the middle comes out clean.

Nutrition information per serving: Kcal: 182, Protein: 4.2g, Carbs: 12.3g, Fats: 14.6g

25. Pineapple Smoothie

Ingredients:

1 cup of pineapple, canned

1 cup of Greek yogurt

½ medium-sized banana, sliced

½ cup of strawberries, halved

1 tsp of vanilla extract

Preparation:

Combine all ingredients in a food processor. Blend until smooth. Add few ice cubes and re-blend. Transfer to a serving glasses and serve immediately.

Nutrition information per serving: Kcal: 122, Protein: 6.3g, Carbs: 24.3g, Fats: 0.8g

26. Rice Yogurt with Fresh Plums and Chia Seeds

Ingredients:

2 tbsp of chia seeds, soaked

½ cup of almond milk

½ cup of rice yogurt

1.5oz quinoa

½ cup of water

2 medium-sized plums, sliced

1 tbsp of honey

Preparation:

Combine the water and almond milk in a medium sized saucepan. Bring it to a boil and add quinoa. Reduce the heat and cook for about 20 minutes, or until all the liquid evaporates.

Transfer the cooked quinoa to a bowl. Stir in the rice yogurt and chia seeds.

Top with sliced plums and serve.

Nutrition information per serving: Kcal: 241, Protein: 4.9g, Carbs: 25g, Fats: 15.8g

27. Rice with Pecans

Ingredients:

10 oz of brown rice

1 small onion, chopped

1 cup of fresh celery, finely chopped

1 medium-sized bell pepper, chopped

2 tbsp of pecans, roughly chopped

1 tbsp of dried sage, ground

2 tbsp of vegetable oil

1 cup of chicken broth, unsalted

12 oz of water

¼ tsp of salt

Preparation:

Combine chicken broth and water in a large pot and bring it to a boil. Add rice and give it a good stir. Reduce the heat to low and cover with a lid. Cook for about 15-20 minutes. remove from the heat and let it stand for 5-6 minutes to cool. Set aside.

Preheat the oil in a large nonstick pan over a low temperature. Add onions and stir-fry until translucent. Stir in the celery and cook for 5 minutes more. Now, add all ingredients except pecans. Add prevoiusly cooked rice and give it a good stir to combine. Cook for 1 minute more. Remove from the heat and serve warm.

Nutrition information per serving: Kcal: 140, Protein: 2.8g, Carbs: 22.3g, Fats: 5.7g

28. Steamed Chicken

Ingredients:

1 lb of chicken legs, cut into bite-sized pieces

¼ tsp of ginger, ground

2 ginger sticks, 2 inches long

1 tbsp of garlic, minced

1 cup of spring onions

¼ tsp of salt

3 tbsp of olive oil

Preparation:

Rub the chicken with ginger and salt. Set aside to marinate for 10 minutes.

Take a large baking sheet and place ginger sticks and garlic at the bottom. Spread the chicken chops evenly over it.

Steam for about 30-35 minutes on high temperature. Remove from the heat to cool completely. Place it into a plastic bags and transfer to cold water.

Now, remove the bones and arange into a serving portion. Meanwhile, combine onions, oil, and a pinch of salt into a mixing bowl. Top over the chicken.

Serve with some cooked vegetables, such as broccoli, cauliflower, etc.

Nutrition information per serving: Kcal: 254, Protein: 26.7g, Carbs: 3.2g, Fats: 15.3g

29. Rice Casserole

Ingredients:

2 large broccoli crowns, chopped

7oz brussel sprouts, halved

1 cup of quinoa, rinsed

4 cups of homemade vegetable broth

2 small onions, finely chopped

1 cup of sour cashew cream

2 tsp dry thyme

4 tbsp of extra virgin olive oil

Salt and pepper to taste

Preparation:

Preheat the oven to 400 degrees.

In a large saucepan, combine quinoa with vegetable broth and dry thyme. Add some salt and pepper to taste and bring it to a boil. Reduce the heat and cook until the liquid is absorbed, about 12-15 minutes. Remove from the heat and set aside.

Heat up the olive oil in a large saucepan. Add onions and stir-fry for 2-3 minutes, or until translucent. Now add chopped broccoli and brussel sprouts. Continue to cook for ten more minutes, or until the broccoli and brussel sprouts are tender-crisp.

Combine the broccoli mixture with quinoa in a large bowl. Add cashew cream and stir well. Place in a lightly oiled shallow casserole dish. Bake for about 20 minutes, or until the top is lightly charred and crisp.

Serve!

Nutrition information per serving: Kcal: 352, Protein: 13g, Carbs: 36.3g, Fats: 18.2g

30. Quinoa Artichoke Soup

Ingredients:

14 oz of artichoke hearts, canned

4 cups od vegetable broth, unsalted

1 cup of white quinoa, pre-cooked

1 small onion, sliced

2 tbsp of fresh lemon juice

1 garlic clove, minced

1 cup of skim milk

1 tsp of brown sugar

¼ tsp of salt

¼ tsp of black pepper, ground

Preparation:

Place quinoa in a large nonstick pan over a medium-high temperature. Cook for 5 minutes, stirring constantly. Remove from the heat and transfer qunioa in another bowl. Reserve the pan.

Preheat the oil in the same pan and add onions and garlic. Stir-fry until translucent. add vegetable broth, lemon juice, and previously toasted quinoa.

Bring it to a boil and redue the temperature to low. Cover with a lid and simmer for 15 minutes, or until tender.

Now, add artichokes and cook for another 5-7 minutes. Remove from the heat and use kitchen hand mixer to puree the soup.

Return the heat and add sugar and milk. Stir constantly for 2 minutes. Remove from the heat and sprinkle with salt and pepper to taste. Serve warm.

Nutrition information per serving: Kcal: 191, Protein: 10.3g, Carbs: 27.4g, Fats: 5.3g

31. Quick Maple Pecan Oatmeal

Ingredients:

2 cups of rolled oats

2 tbsp of coconut flour

½ cup of pecans, roughly chopped

3 tbsp of raisins, chopped

3 tbsp of maple syrup

1 tbsp of honey

1 tsp of cinnamon, ground

1 tsp of vanilla extract

Preparation:

Use package instructions to cook oats. Remove from the heat and let it cool. Transfer to a large bowl and add all other ingredients.

Stir all well to combine and serve wiht some extra nuts if you like.

Nutrition information per serving: Kcal: 313, Protein: 5.6g, Carbs: 63.5g, Fats: 3.6g

32. Asparagus and Leek Soup

Ingredients:

1 lb of fresh wild asparagus, trimmed and chopped

1 cup of leeks, chopped

2 cups of vegetable broth, unstalted

2 medium-sized potatoes, peeled and chopped

2 garlic cloves, minced

1 tbsp of olive oil

½ cup of green beans, pre-cooked

1 tbsp of fresh parsley, finely chopped

2 cups of skim milk

¼ tsp of lemon juice

¼ tsp of salt

¼ tsp of black pepper, ground

Preparation:

Preheat the oil in a large skillet over a medium-low temperature. Add leeks and cook for about 5-7 minutes, or until soften. Add garlic and cook for another minute. Stir constantly.

Pour in the vegetable broth. Increase the temperature to high and add potatoes. Cover with a lid and cook until potatoes are fork-tender. Add asparagus and green beans. Cook for another 4-5 minutes. remove from the heat and stir in all other ingredients. Stir all well and transfer to a food processor or blender. Blend until nicely smooth creamy mixture. Return the mixture to the skillet.

Cook for 15 minutes on low heat and remove from the heat. Let it cool and serve.

Nutrition information per serving: Kcal: 190, Protein: 8.7g, Carbs: 28.8g, Fats: 4.7g

33. Sweet Rice Noodles

Ingredients:

14oz rice noodles

2 tbsp of olive oil

2 tsp ground turmeric

2 cups of coconut milk

½ cup of sour cashew cream

2 tbsp of almond butter

¼ cup of fresh lime juice

A handful of toasted cashews

1 tsp of powdered honey

1 medium-sized onion, finely chopped

1 tbsp fresh ginger, grated

Preparation:

Soak the noodles for five minutes. Drain and set aside.

Heat up the olive oil and add ground turmeric. Briefly cook for about a minute. Now add coconut milk and bring it to a boil. Reduce the heat and add almond butter, cashew craem, fresh lime juice, cashews, honey, chopped onion, and fresh ginger. Continue to cook for about five minutes.

Add noodles and mix well. Cover and allow it to warm up. Serve.

Nutrition information per serving: Kcal: 342, Protein: 3.9g, Carbs: 24.7g, Fats: 27g

34. Ice Cappuccino Smoothie

Ingredients:

1 tsp of instant espresso powder

1 tbsp of liquid chocolate

1 cup of skim milk

¼ tsp of cinnamon

1 tsp of honey

Preparation:

Combine all ingredients in a blender except cinnamon. Blend until smooth. Add few ice cubes, and re-blend. Transfer to a serving glass. Sprinkle with cinnamon and serve.

Nutrition information per serving: Kcal: 169, Protein: 8.7g, Carbs: 24.3g, Fats: 3.1g

35. Almond Yogurt with Nuts

Ingredients:

1 cup of almond yogurt

A handful of walnuts, chopped

1 tbsp of chia seeds

1 tbsp of homemade fig spread

Preparation:

Combine one cup of almond yogurt with chia seeds. Top with chopped nuts and fig spread. Serve immediately!

Nutrition information per serving: Kcal: 192, Protein: 6.1g, Carbs: 33g, Fats: 7.9g

36. Spring Purple Salad

Ingredients:

½ medium red cabbage head

2 large spring onions, sliced

2 medium-sized carrots, sliced

¼ cup of extra virgin olive oil

2 tbsp of fresh lemon juice

½ tsp of sea salt

½ tsp of freshly ground black pepper

Preparation:

Cut cabbage in large pieces and place it in a food processor. Pulse quickly until chopped roughly. Be careful not to process too much.

Combine the cabbage with sliced carrots and spring onions. Toss with olive oil, lemon juice, sea salt, and black pepper.

Nutrition information per serving: Kcal: 254, Protein: 1.1g, Carbs: 8.5g, Fats: 25.4g

37. Rosemary Couscous

Ingredients:

1 cup of instant couscous

2 large carrots

½ tsp of dried rosemary

1 cup of green beans, cooked and drained

10 green olives, pitted

1 tbsp of lemon juice

1 tbsp of orange juice

1 tbsp of orange zest

4 tbsp of olive oil

½ tsp of salt

Preparation:

Wash and peel carrots. Cut into thin slices. Heat up 2 tbsp of olive oil in a large pan over medium heat.

Add carrots and cook, stirring constantly. It should be tender after about 10-15 minutes. Add rosemary, green beans, olives and orange juice. Mix well.

Continue to cook and stir occasionally.

Combine lemon juice with 1 cup of water. Add this mixture to a saucepan and mix with 2 tbsp of olive oil, orange zest and salt. Allow it to boil and add couscous. Remove from heat and allow it to stand for about 15 minutes.

Pour these two mixtures into a large bowl and mix well with a tablespoon.

Nutrition information per serving: Kcal: 396, Protein: 1.8g, Carbs: 12.9g, Fats: 28g

38. Lean Grilled Avocado

Ingredients:

1 large avocado, chopped

¼ cup of water

1 tbsp of ground curry

2 tbsp of olive oil

1 tbsp of tomato sauce

1 tsp of chopped parsley

¼ tsp of red pepper

¼ tsp of sea salt

Preparation:

Heat up olive oil in a large saucepan, over a medium temperature. In a small bowl, combine ground curry, tomato sauce, chopped parsley, red pepper and sea salt. Add water and cook for about 5 minutes, over a medium temperature.

Add chopped avocado, stir well and cook for another few minutes, until all the liquid evaporates. Turn off the heat and cover.

Let it stand for about 15-20 minutes before serving.

Nutrition information per serving: Kcal: 332, Protein: 2.2g, Carbs: 10.2g, Fats: 33g

39. Turkey Cauliflower Omelet

Ingredients:

1 lb of turkey breast, boneless and skinless

2 lbs of cauliflower, grated

4 garlic cloves, crushed

3 large eggs

1 cup of spring onions, chopped

4 tbsp of olive oil

¼ tsp of sea salt

¼ tsp of black pepper, ground

Preparation:

Squeeze the excessive liquid out of cauliflower and transfer to a large bowl. Set aside.

Preheat the oil in a large saucepan over a medium-high temperature. Add garlic and stir-fry until translucent. Add meat and cook until for about 10-15 minutes, or until almost set. Reduce the heat to low.

Meanwhile, beat the eggs in a mixing bowl nad pour into a saucepan. Stir in grated cauliflower. Add a pinch of salt and pepper to taste. Cook until eggs scrambled, or until cauliflower tender crisp.

Spoon the spring onion and spread over the meat. Cook for another minute and remove from the heat. Add extra salt if necessarry.

Serve warm.

Nutrition information per serving: Kcal: 361, Protein: 29.3g, Carbs: 20.1g, Fats: 19.3g

40. Baked Mushrooms in Tomato Sauce

Ingredients:

1 cup of button mushrooms

1 large tomato

3 tbsp of olive oil

2 cloves of garlic

1 tbsp of fresh basil

salt and pepper to taste

Preparation:

Wash and peel tomato. Cut in small pieces. Chop garlic and mix with tomato and fresh basil. Heat up the olive oil in a saucepan and put tomato in it. Add ¼ cup of water, mix well and cook for about 15 minutes, on a low temperature, until the water evaporates. Stir constantly. After about 15 minutes, when all the water has evaporated, remove from heat.

Wash and drain mushrooms. Place them in small baking dish and spread tomato sauce over it. Salt and pepper to taste.

Preheat the oven to 300 degrees and bake for about 10-15 minutes.

Nutrition information per serving: Kcal: 209, Protein: 2.1g, Carbs: 5.8g, Fats: 21.4g

41. Sour potato soup

Ingredients:

1 large potato, peeled and chopped into bite-sized pieces

1 medium-sized onion, peeled and finely chopped

2 small carrots, sliced

4 cups of vegetable broth

A handful of fresh parsley

1 tbsp of apple cider vinegar

1 tsp of salt

½ tsp of pepper

2 tbsp extra virgin olive oil

Preparation:

Heat up the oil in a heavy bottomed saucepan. Add onions and stir-fry until translucent. Now add sliced carrot and potatoes. Continue to cook for five more minutes.

Pour in the vegetable broth, add apple cider, salt, and pepper. Reduce the heat to minimum and cook until potatoes are fork tender.

Serve warm.

Nutrition information per serving: Kcal: 192, Protein: 7.2g, Carbs: 22.3, Fats: 8.5g

42. Mushroom Salad with Gorgonzola

Ingredients:

1 lb of button mushrooms, chopped

4 oz of Gorgonzola cheese, crumbled

1 bell pepper, roasted, finely chopped

1 cup of Romaine lettuce, chopped

1 cup of sour cream

1 tbsp of mayonnaise

1 tbsp of balsamic vinegar

1 garlic clove, minced

1 tbsp of butter

¼ tsp of salt

¼ tsp of black pepper, ground

Preparation:

Combine cheese, sour cream, vinegar, mayonnaise, red pepper, and garlic in a large mixing bowl. Mash well with fork or use an electric mixer. Sprinkle with some salt and pepper and set aside to allow flavors to mingle.

Melt the butter in a large frying pan over a medium-high temperature. Add mushrooms and cook for 10 minutes, or until set. Stir occasionally. Remove from the heat.

Place a handful of lettuce on a serving plate and spoon the previously made cheese mixture. Top with mushrooms and serve.

Nutrition information per serving: Kcal: 298, Protein: 12.1g, Carbs: 11.9g, Fats: 24.6g

43. Tuna Stuffed Eggplant

Ingredients:

1 lb of tuna steaks, skinless and boneless

2 medium-sized eggplants, halved

3 tbsp of caper, drained

1 tbsp of olive oil

½ tbsp of butter, melted

2 tbsp of fresh basil, finely chopped

¼ tsp of salt

Preparation:

Preheat the oven to 370°F.

Combine tuna, butter, and capers in a food processor. Blend until smooth and transfer to a medium bowl. Stir in the basil and set aside.

Take a large baking sheet and place some baking paper. Spread the eggplant halves onto it and sprinkle with some olive oil. Put it in the oven and bake until eggplants are fork-tender. remove from the heat and let it cool for 10 minutes.

Spoon the tuna mixture into each eggplant. Sprinkle with salt to taste. Top with extra capers or grated cheese. Serve.

Nutrition information per serving: Kcal: 322, Protein: 36.1g, Carbs: 16.3g, Fats: 12.6g

44. Sour Boiled Eggs

Ingredients:

2 medium onions

4 boiled eggs

1 cup of chopped pickles

1 tsp of grated fresh ginger

1 tbsp of low fat cream

1 tbsp of lemon juice

1 tbsp of olive oil

1 tsp of ground turmeric

salt to taste

Preparation:

Peel and cut the onions. Salt it and leave it to stand for about 5 minutes. Wash and squeeze, and sprinkle some lemon juice over it and leave it.

Add the eggs to a pot of boiling water. Be very gentle while doing this to prevent the eggs to crack.

One useful tip to prepare the perfect eggs is to add 1 tbsp of baking soda into the boiling water. This will make a peeling process much easier.

Boil the eggs for 8 minutes. You can use a kitchen timer, or simply your watch. After 8 minutes, drain the water and place the eggs under the cold water for few minutes. Peel and slice the eggs.

Combine it with chopped pickles and ginger. Add onions and season with olive oil, low fat cream, salt and turmeric. Serve cold.

Nutrition information per serving: Kcal: 247, Protein: 12.8g, Carbs: 14.2g, Fats: 16.2g

45.Kiwi Banana Smoothie

Ingredients:

2 medium-sized kiwi, peeled

1 large banana, sliced

1 tbsp of lemon juice

½ cup of Greek yogurt

1 tbsp of honey

Preparation:

Combine all ingredients in a food processor. Blend until smooth. Add few ice cubes and re-blend for 30 seconds. Transfer the mixture to a serving glasess. Top with extra honey for sweetness.

Nutrition information per serving: Kcal: 178, Protein: 6.7g, Carbs: 37.5g, Fats: 1.7g

46. Shrimps in Tomato Sauce with Potatoes

Ingredients:

12 oz of shrimps, peeled and deveined

4 small potatoes, peeled and halved

2 tbsp of heavy cream

4 tbsp of Parmesan cheese, grated

1 tsp of oregano

2 tbsp of olive oil

2 medium-sized tomatoes, blended

¼ tsp of salt

¼ tsp of black pepper, ground

Preparation:

Place potatoes in a large pot over a medium-high temperature. Sprinkle with salt to taste and cook until fork-tender. Remove from the heat and drain. Set aside.

Meanwhile, place tomatoes in blender and blend until smooth. Set aside.

Preheat the oil in a large nonstick skillet over a medium-high temperature. add shrimps and tomato mixture. Stir well and cook for about 5-6 minutes or until set. Add heavy cream and cheese and give it a good stir. Cook until cheese melts. Remove from the heat and let it cool for a while.

Place potatoes into a serving plate. Spoon the shrimp sauce on top. Sprinkle with oregano to taste and serve.

Nutrition information per serving: Kcal: 317, Protein: 23.1g, Carbs: 30.8g, Fats: 11.6g

47. Cucumber Quinoa Berry Salad

Ingredients:

1 large cucumber, sliced

1 cup of white quinoa, pre-cooked

1 cup of fresh cranberries

1 cup of fresh blueberries

2 tbsp of almonds, roughly chopped

1 small red onion, diced

1 tsp of maple syrup

1 tbsp of olive oil

2 tbsp of balsamic vinegar

Preparation:

Place quinoa in a large pot. Pour enough water to cover it. Bring it to a boil and then reduce the temperature to low. Cook for about 13-15 minutes and remove from the heat. Fluff with spoon and transfer to a large bowl. Set aside to cool for a while.

Meanwhile, combine oil, vinegar, and maple syrup. Whisk well to combine and pour it over the quinoa.

Now, add cucumbers, onion and fruits and give it a good stir. Set aside or refrigerate for 20 minutes before serving.

Nutrition information per serving: Kcal: 171, Protein: 4.7g, Carbs: 30.4g, Fats: 4.3g

48. Mixed Berries Pancakes

Ingredients:

3 eggs

½ cup coconut flour

½ cup almond flour

1 cup of coconut milk

1 tsp of apple vinegar

1 tsp vanilla, minced

½ tsp of baking soda

¼ tsp salt

coconut oil for frying

3 cups of mixed fresh berries

Preparation:

In a large bowl, combine the coconut flour, almond flour, minced vanilla, baking soda, and salt. In a smaller bowl, mix coconut milk and apple vinegar. Whisk in the coconut mixture until smooth dough.

Using a nonstick skillet, heat up the coconut oil over a medium heat. Spread the desired amount of dough over the skillet. Use a spoon to smooth the surface of each pancake. Fry for about 2-3 minutes on each side.

Top with mixed fresh berries and 1 tbsp of agave syrup.

Nutrition information per serving: Kcal: 186, Protein: 11.9g, Carbs: 55g, Fats: 19.5g

49. Banana Raisins Cookies

Ingredients:

1 large banana, sliced

¼ cup of dried raisins

1 ½ cup of all-purpose flour

½ tsp of baking powder

1 cup of rolled oats

1 tsp of baking soda

2 tbsp of butter

1 large egg

3 tbsp of honey

1 tsp of vanilla extract

½ cup of dark chocolate, finely chopped

2 tbsp of walnuts, roughly chopped

¼ tsp of salt

Preparation:

Preheat the oven to 375°F.

Combine flour, baking soda, and baking powder in a large bowl. Mix well with a spoon and add honey, butter, salt, banana, and vanilla. Use a hand mixer to combine and mix until you get thick batter. Form the cookies with hands and roll into the rolled oats, chocolate chops, raisins, and walnuts.

Line some parchment paper over a baking sheet and spread the cookies. Make 1 inch space between the cookies. Put it in the oven and bake for about 10-15 minutes or until golden brown and crisp. Remove from the heat and set aside to cool before serving.

Nutrition information per serving: Kcal: 562, Protein: 10.3g, Carbs: 90.2g, Fats: 17.5g

50. Rice Pilaf with Spinach

Ingredients:

1 cup of brown rice, pre-cooked, drained and rinsed

1 lb of fresh spinach, pre-cooked

1 garlic clove, minced

1 small onion, diced

1 tbsp of vegetable oil

1 tsp of dried thyme, ground

¼ cup of cheddar cheese, shredded

2 large eggs

Preparation:

Preheat the oven to 350°F.

Place rice in a large pot and pour water enough to cover it. Cook for 30 minutes or until almost done. Remove from the heat. Drain and rinse few times with cold water. Set aside.

Place spinach in the same pot and pour enough water to cover it. Cook until until soften. Remove from the heat and set aside.

Preheat the oil in the same pot and add onion andgarlic. Stir-fry until translucent and remove from the heat.

Now, combine pre-cooked rice and spinach, cheese, and thyme in a large mixing bowl. Beat the egg into the bowl and give it a good stir to combine. Sprinkle a pinch of salt to taste and set aside.

Grease a nonstick baking sheet and spread the mixture evenly. Cover with aluminu foil and put it in the oven. Bake for about 20-25 minutes. Remove the foil, and bake for another 5-6 minutes. Remove from the heat and make 4 equal portions.

You can top with one tablespoon of sour cream. However, this is optional.

Nutrition information per serving: Kcal: 301, Protein: 12.2g, Carbs: 42.3g, Fats: 10.3g

51. Trout with Veggies

Ingredients:

2 lbs of trout fillet, boneless

1 medium-sized tomato, wedged

1 medium-sized bell pepper, cut into strips

1 small onion, sliced

3 tbsp of lemon juice

3 tbsp of cilantro, chopped

1 tsp of rosemary, finely chopped

¼ tsp of sea salt

¼ tsp of black pepper, ground

Preparation:

Preheat oven to 350 °F.

Wash, pat dry, and place the filets in a large greased baking dish.

Combine tomato, pepper, onion, lemon juice, cilantro, salt, and pepper in a mixing bowl. Stir well and spoon the mixture over the fillets. Place it in the oven and bake for 20 minutes, or until fish fork-tender.

Nutrition information per serving: Kcal: 305, Protein: 34.2g, Carbs: 4.3, Fats: 11.4g

52. Potato Salad

Ingredients:

3 lbs large potatoes, pre-cooked

1 cup of fresh celery, chopped

½ cup of spring onions, chopped

¼ cup of sour cream

½ cup of cottage cheese, crumbled

1 tbsp of lemon juice

1 tsp of apple cider vinegar

½ tbsp of yellow mustard

¼ tsp of salt

¼ tsp of black pepper, ground

Preparation:

Place potaotes in a pot of boiling water and cook until fork-tender. drain and set aside to cool.

Combine potatoes, spring onions, celery, parsley, and green onions in a large bowl. Set aside.

Meanwhile, combine sour cream, lemon juice, vinegar, mustard, salt, and pepper in a food processor. Blend until smooth and pour over the previously prepared salad. Refrigerate for 1 hour before serving.

Nutrition information per serving: Kcal: 302, Protein: 9.8g, Carbs: 57.1, Fats: 4.2g

ADDITIONAL TITLES FROM THIS AUTHOR

70 Effective Meal Recipes to Prevent and Solve Being Overweight: Burn Fat Fast by Using Proper Dieting and Smart Nutrition

By

Joe Correa CSN

48 Acne Solving Meal Recipes: The Fast and Natural Path to Fixing Your Acne Problems in Less Than 10 Days!

By

Joe Correa CSN

41 Alzheimer's Preventing Meal Recipes: Reduce or Eliminate Your Alzheimer's Condition in 30 Days or Less!

By

Joe Correa CSN

70 Effective Breast Cancer Meal Recipes: Prevent and Fight Breast Cancer with Smart Nutrition and Powerful Foods

By

Joe Correa CSN

www.ingramcontent.com/pod-product-compliance
Lightning Source LLC
Chambersburg PA
CBHW051033030426
42336CB00015B/2847